Setting the Perfect

hair goals

The Natural's Black Book to Recipes, Rituals, & Round-Ups

#hairgoalsblackbook

hairgoalsblackbook.com

LEGAL DISCLAIMER

Kim Harris KIM XI LEGACY ENTERPRISE LLC ©2017 - All rights reserved.

All trademarks and brands within this book are owned by KIM XI LEGACY ENTERPRISE LLC.

Disclaimer and Terms of Use

The Author and Publisher has strived to be as accurate and complete as possible in the creation of this book, notwithstanding the fact that she does not warrant or represent at any time that the contents within are accurate due to the rapidly changing nature of the Internet. While all attempts have been made to verify information provided in this publication, the Author and Publisher assumes no responsibility for errors, omissions, or contrary interpretation of the subject matter herein.

Any perceived slights of specific persons, peoples, or organizations are unintentional. In practical advice books, like anything else in life, there are no guarantees of results. Readers are cautioned to rely on their own judgment about their individual circumstances and act accordingly.

This book is not intended for use as a source of hair care advice. All readers are advised to seek services of competent professionals in the hair care industry and fields.

Contents

About Kim

Sharing information has always been my passion, no matter the topic – if it helps others to have, do, and be better – I share it!

I'm asked all the time when out, "what do you do to make your hair grow?" I always answer, "the better question would be – what do I do to get it healthy and stay on my head!".

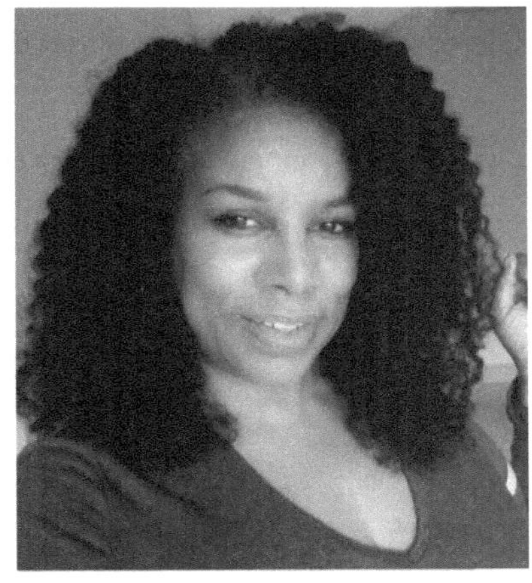

November 2017 Selfie – Two-strand twist out.

My healthy hair reflects who I am and how I feel which is FANTASTIC!

It all began with setting perfect hair goals for my hair.

My natural hair journey took me for an emotional loop, but once I began to embrace it and feel the authenticity it delivered, I realized that I could not be the only one who has experienced this. So, I wanted to share what I have learned about my natural locks and bring all the resources that helped me along the way to you.

This is your little black book that you can refer to when you don't have hours to spend watching videos or searching online. This will give you a good, solid starting point.

In 2010, I decided to rid myself of perms forever. I officially started my hair journey in April 2013, three years after a massive hair fall that scared the crap out of me.

It took a minute (figuratively) to feel what my hair was allowing me to feel – liberated. Unchained from society's view of what was considered beautiful.   The transition was tough, but I stumbled my way through, and with no regrets.

My hair required special attention because of my 50+ status and my ever-changing biological composition. Once I got that under wraps, all was well in the hair world! ☺

There are some processes that will not work for you, others will. Be focused, diligent, patient, and well-informed about what your hair needs are and creating your perfect hair goals will be easy.

Stay Natural...Stay Beautiful!

--- Kim

So, It Begins...

Natural hair - chemically-free and allowed to do its own natural thang!

Women around the world are embracing their authentic natural hair. Breaking the bondage of years of chemical abuse, trying to fit into a mold that was not designed for them in the first place.

When I was a young girl, the boys went crazy for the girl with the long hair. When I became a young woman, the men drooled at a Black woman with long *straight* hair. During that time, there was not a market for "weaves" or "sew ins" - it truly was our own hair.   When you watch old episodes of SOUL TRAIN back in the early 70's, it was just one Big Afro after another. Those who had straight hair were either Caucasian, "Mixed", or could afford to get a permanent relaxer on a regular basis. Everyone else, like me, struggled to each week to blow dry, hot comb, and flat-iron until I could achieve that *long silky* look.

My gene-pool predisposed me for long, thick hair. However, straight hair wasn't in the cards for me. And like millions of naturals, I labored for hours washing and blow drying this forest on my head to appear more "acceptable" in society.

Eventually, I did what millions of other women of color with kinky hair did -- I permed it! It served its purpose until it didn't anymore. My problem with relaxers didn't show up until after many years of use; and, when my body was going through hormonal changes my hair became symptomatic with breakage and excessive hair fall.

I realized that if I didn't find a solution quickly, I would be like one of millions of women who have irreversible bald patches, and I did not want that. So, I made the courageous decision to nix the relaxers forever.

I did not opt for the BIG CHOP. Instead, I nursed my hair through the transition as best I could, knowing that over time there would be some severe breakage. I was not wrong. My hair took at least 2 years to get to the point where the new growth was strong enough to bare the journey of growing out the perm the rest of the way.

I trimmed the remaining two inches of perm out of my hair and that is when my official natural hair journey began - April 2013.

I searched for products that were designed for my hair type, "natural", and I could not find anything that worked. I started experimenting with DIY, because I figured that Mother Nature wouldn't hurt me, and it was probably healthier than what I bought in the store. But still, there were serious holes in my hair care regimen and I was strictly in survival mode with my hair.

One of the first resources I found online for natural hair care was JUST NATURAL HAIR CARE. I was amazed at the quality of their products and started on a regimen of strengthening my strands. This was the break I was looking for, and my hair showed significant improvement.

I did more research on hair loss in women and found that aging plays a big factor in the growth and health of hair. I have cited articles in the RESOURCES section of this book. When I discovered what my own issues were with hormones, I found healthy, bio-identical solutions to balance my hormonal system. This was a huge factor in getting my hair back to health. I strongly recommend that if you're 40+, you have a hormone panel done at your next doctor's appointment.

My hair journey has had some successes, fails, and setbacks. But, now I feel that my hair is healthier and stronger than ever. I realize that my hair ritual is more spiritual than anything because it connects me with the essence of who I am more profoundly. It brings me to the most authentic expression of myself, and when I'm in that space, I am liberated and give more freely to the world.

Every week, I go through the ritual of caring for my hair in a very routine way, so as not to disturb its intention of health and growth. I'm consciously aware of how comforting it is to care for my hair in a loving way and deliberately choose only what will optimize its function.

Some of the most interesting conversations with myself arise out of this intimate time together with my hair. This intimacy is what makes my natural hair journey *spiritual.* It's real, this journey of self-discovery; unfolding new aspects of my thoughts about life and my role in it.

Every natural I have ever spoken with has confirmed this renewed sense of self with liberating their locks.

As an African-American woman, I grew up with the reinforced belief that my hair is my crown, that each strand is a precious jewel that if lost, could not be replaced. Somewhere along the way, I buried that belief and became subjugated with false images of myself.

Not fully understanding the magnitude of what I was doing, I used chemicals, dyes, and heating tools that damaged and weakened my strands. And as life would have it, the aging process brought a whole other set of challenges when it came to my hair care and retention.

In this book, I share the DIY recipes, rituals, and resources that helped me to find my way back to healthy natural hair. It would be selfish of me to take full credit for my hair journey success, because as with any journey, guides are necessary to help you reach your final goal. Mine were found in the world of social media, YouTube® to be exact.

Like so many naturals, or even those who want to transition to natural, I did not know where to begin. I simply went to YouTube® and consumed videos like crazy on the topic of *Natural Hair Care*. I understand that everyone doesn't have time to do that; some work, have children or spouses, or just have a life.

Of all the thousands of hours of videos I have viewed over the years, only a hand full of natural hair influencers gave me the inspiration to take my natural hair journey seriously. And as a result, my hair is stronger, healthier, and more beautiful than I can ever remember. I share some of the inspired recipes which were modified for my specific hair type that helped the process of maintaining healthy hair easier.

The *Round-Up* of superstar influencers featured in this book are authentic, share quantifiable value on their channels, and reminds us all to embrace our natural hair. They inspired me to take the initiative to experiment with nature and discover new and exciting ways to get my curls back to health and behave flawlessly.

Once you begin your own journey, you will find that you, too, will tweak and modify recipes and treatments along the way.

When you find your *rhythm* in your own journey, you will fall in love with your hair and yourself, all over again!

YOUR HAIR JOURNEY IS YOURS ALONE – SO, LET IT BEGIN...

CAUTIONARY TALES

Our natural hair requires us to look at the chemistry, biological, and genetical make up more closely.

We live in an information overload world, and sometimes we just are not aware of what is beneficial to our own well-being because we are receiving too much of it and are often confused by it.

When it comes to information about our hair, we are inundated through millions of videos, blogs, and social media feeds, all vying for our attention. Product pushes, recommendations, testimonials, and demonstrations. It's so easy to get sucked in and want to buy everything you just learned about, thinking it will somehow provide the same results you just witnessed.

Maybe that works, and maybe it doesn't.

Hair is responsive, and based on its type and condition will respond to whatever we apply to it. Someone who was born with fine hair may not be able to use the heavier creams or oils that I like to use on my hair. It will respond differently.

Someone who uses a store-bought conditioner or curl cream and has beautiful definition in their curls, may not work for me.

There are some ingredients that have adverse effects on all kinky, curly, coily hair no matter how much they are advertised as being beneficial.

For example, silicone is used in most conditioners. Its chemical composition makes the hair feel soft and smooth while wet. However, when natural hair dries with conditioner containing silicone, the hair becomes more brittle and breaks easily.

When silicone conditioners are combined with the use of alcohol-based gels, there can be severe breakage, if not careful.

It is important to read the labels of products you purchase. Water should be in the first three ingredients. If silicone appears in the first five ingredients, consider another product. Review the articles in the RESOURCES section of this book.

Look for labels that read:
> **NO Sulfates, Parabens, Phthalates, Paraffin, Propylene Glycol, Mineral Oil, Silicones [See RESOURCES for article on Silicones], Synthetic color or fragrances, DEA, and NO Animal Testing.**

Some great brands that are highly recommended and rendered safe and nourishing for your hair care needs are:

Shea Moisture	**Just Natural Skincare**
Curls	**Mielle Organics**
Puracy	**Cantu**
Oyin Handmade	

Too much of anything is not good, but too much of the wrong thing can be detrimental. Your hair does not need a lot of product to remain healthy.

Choose a few of the essential products like cleanser, conditioner, and daily moisturizer to stock your pantry. Then, add a specialized treatment for strengthening, like a protein treatment.

One final thing; be careful of the frequency in which protein is applied to your hair. It is a strengthening application, too much can cause your hair to become brittle and break easily.

CROWNING GLORY

The year is 2009. The moment of realization hit me like a ton of bricks. Standing in the bathroom after washing my hair and taking the blow dryer to it, a flush of panic raced through my veins when I looked down and around my feet were clumps of freshly broken strands. There was a problem and I didn't know what to do about it. So, like anyone else who is in a state of shock and denial, I simply ignored it...panic and all!

My crown was fading, and fading fast. Once I realized that the hair fall was not a flux, I decided to do something about it. So, I glued myself to the internet looking for information of every kind concerning hair loss in women. I made some startling discoveries and as a result found information that guided me to change my hair habits and embrace my natural side.

For years, I had permed my hair every six to eight weeks without fail. I colored it at least twice a year. I rarely performed any kind of protein treatment. However, I did have the wherewithal to condition, occasionally. This routine was having a serious impact on my hair. To add to the devastation of hair fall were the symptoms of para-menopause, which I did not learn about until several years later. I knew I could fix this before it was too late. This was my crown and I was not going to lose it!

The world we live in always begs us to have it "now". So, anything that appears to give us instant gratification, we jump all over it. We follow the crowd instead of creating our own way.

Well, let me be frank...
The quest for long, healthy, kinky, curly, or coily natural hair is riddled with trial and error. Our ancestors knew that Mother Nature was, and still is, the best remedy for curing what ails us.

They were patient in preparing concoctions that implored the earth's wisdom through herbs and plants.

The hair goal priority is <u>always</u> healthy hair first. Healthy hair results in consistent growth because there is less breakage and harm done to the hair.

This movement to embrace what is natural to us – our natural hair - is not a fad. Our hair is our most visual representation of our strength: *spiritual, mental, and physical.* It doesn't matter whether it's short or long.

TRANSITIONING HAIR

On average, the human scalp has anywhere from 100,000 to 150,000 hair follicles. According to WebMD, it's typical to lose roughly 100 hairs each day. As you get older, your hair begins to grow at a slower rate. Even if you're losing an average amount, it takes longer for new hairs to appear, which can contribute to the appearance of thinning or bald spots. <From <https://www.creditdonkey.com/hair-loss-statistics.html>

According to Anabel Kingsley, a leading Trichologist at the Philip Kingsley Clinic in London, there are two types of hair loss:

Genetic:
There's a chance you're genetically predisposed to hair thinning, which means you may see a progressive, gradual reduction in hair volume. "In these instances, certain hair follicles are sensitive to male hormones – and this sensitivity causes follicles to gradually shrink and produce slightly finer and shorter hairs with each passing hair growth cycle." Explains Anabel.

Reactive:
This means your hair loss is the result of a trigger. "Excessive daily hair shedding (which is known as telogen effluvium) is not reliant on having a genetic predisposition, it occurs as the result of an internal imbalance or upset, such as a nutritional deficiency, severe stress, crash dieting or an illness" says Anabel. From <http://www.cosmopolitan.com/uk/beauty-hair/advice/a48958/hair-loss-reasons/>

Hair loss in women is largely attributed to hormonal imbalance, as it is in men and is one of the lesser known and less common menopause symptoms. Hair loss in women increases during para-menopause and menopause because androgens, namely dihydrotestosterone (DHT), is more prevalent than estrogen. Other hormonal imbalances such as thyroid problems

and genetic hormonal responses to autoimmune conditions can also cause thinning of the hair and premature balding in women.
From <https://www.bodylogicmd.com/for-women/hair-loss?tid=cpc.google.g.search_symptom.hair_loss_women.%2Bh air%20loss%20%2Bwomen.b.c.{adid}.1406756188&gclid=CjwKC AiA1O3RBRBHEiwAq5fD_PRqTF6Dg9UFrVHgxWaELmpe2NX8O WHybExkqlrAM3hqDiqNptO4vRoC1CUQAvD_BwE>

Transitioning from chemically treated to its natural state can cause tremendous stress and trauma to your strands. Your hair will respond by acting similarly to someone who experiences withdrawal symptoms from an addictive substance. It will begin to break, misbehave, not style properly, and fall out. Basically, give you a headache and make you want to abandon the natural journey ship altogether.

Hang in there!

Don't give up just yet ~ there are some things that you may be overlooking.

Assess where you are in your life to see if there are some other things you can do to aid in the transition. Consider your age, environment, diet, mental health.

Ask yourself these questions:

What types of foods are you eating?

Are you taking vitamin supplements?

Is your body deficient in any key nutrients for hair health?

Have you begun para-menopause (usually begins around age 35) or are you in menopause (usually around age 50), or post-menopause (around age 55+)?

Are you stressed?

When you address some of these and other areas of your life, you can improve your hair's health and ease your journey to natural.

One of the biggest changes I made in my own personal journey was diet. I became more conscious of the food I was eating throughout the day and made subtle changes along the way.

For example, I eat more green, leafy vegetables, drink more water, and increased my fruit intake considerably. I don't eat any fried foods, and I made my groceries list at least 90% USDA Organic.

Not everyone will follow that pattern, and that's okay. You do you!

Remember, hair is only *alive* at the scalp, the hair shaft is dead. The hair derives its nutrients from the body through the scalp. The mistake most naturals make is thinking that topical solutions alone will nourish the hair. That is only partially true. A topical solution that absorbs into the hair shaft is most beneficial to strengthening the hair. Another factor to consider is maintaining a healthy pH balance. Excess product can throw off the balance and result in product build up. The rigorous routines you put your hair through to remove that build up causes extra stress on the strands resulting in breakage.

Bottom-line…what you put in your body will be fed through the hair follicle to the shaft providing the most effective distribution of nutrients to the hair. Healthy eating habits show up in beautiful, strong, shiny locks!

BEST METHOD

The L.O.C. and the L.C.O. method was a little confusing to decipher at first. Many people think they are the same. The application of the products {depending on how you interpret the acronym} can affect your hair differently. It refers to the moisture retention process after washing your hair.

Depending on who you watch or listen to, the L.O.C. acronym could mean different things. Some refer to the "L" as *leave-In*, others as *liquid.* For this book, and my own personal use, the 'L' stands for *liquid.*

The same with the "C" - some refer to it as *conditioner*, others as *crème.* Again, for this book and my own personal use, the 'C' stands for crème.

The method you choose will be based on what you know about your own curl pattern and porosity. I use the L.C.O. method for my type 4 hair.

Liquid
The liquid can be plain distilled water, or a spritz [see RECIPES] used to keep hair moist, but not too wet while detangling and twisting.

Crème
Depending on your hair density, type, and porosity, you will want to choose a crème that works best. For thicker strands, thicker density, using a heavier crème is better. For thinner strands, thick density, using a lighter crème in smaller sections is better. For thinner strands, thin density, use a very light butter. For thin hair, use lights oils that absorb into the cuticle more easily are Avocado Oil, Sesame Oil, and Coconut Oil.

The Mango Delight Butter recipe in the RECIPE section has been modified to suit my hair. It can also be modified to your hair needs. It provides nutrients and fatty acids to the hair to keep the strand flexible.

Oil
Use an oil that absorbs into the cuticle of the strands. Coconut, Avocado, and Sesame are best. The hair growth oil in RECIPES can also be used to seal it all in. If you are planning on wearing a twist out, use the Flaxseed Gel for added definition and hold. (See RECIPES)

You may find that the L.O.C. method works best for your hair type and condition. I recommend trying both to see which one your hair responds to more favorably. You can tell when your hair retains moisture longer than usual.

For great videos on the science of the L.C.O. and L.O.C. method, check out **Green Beauty** on YouTube®.

Natural RECIPES

Ayurvedic DIY

HENNA MASK

1/2 cup Henna
1/2 cup Aloe Vera Powder
1/4 cup Fenugreek Powder
1 TBSP Avocado Oil

Mix all ingredients with room temperature or warm water until the consistency of a pancake batter.

Apply to freshly washed hair that has been detangled and sectioned.

Once applied, cover in a plastic cap, and leave in for 1-2 hours. Rinse with warm water.

Optional:
You can apply conditioner (not deep conditioner) for manageability. Rinse cool water.

Style as usual.

This is a modified recipe inspired by YouTube® Influencer, **Curly Proverbz.**

Butters DIY

MANGO DELIGHT BUTTER

Butters
1/3 cup Mango Butter
2 TBSP Avocado Butter
2 TBSP Cupuacu Butter
2 TBSP Cocoa Butter
2 TBSP Jojoba Butter

Oils
1 tsp. Argan Oil
1/8 tsp. Vitamin E Oil
1 tsp. Grapeseed Oil
1 tsp. Castor Oil (Hexane-free)
1/4 tsp. Sweet Almond Oil

Aloe Vera Plant, cubed, blended and strained or
1/4 cup Aloe Vera Juice or 2 TBSP Aloe Vera Gel

1. Melt all butter in double boiler on <u>low heat.</u> You don't want to cook the butters, just melt them.
2. Stir until they are melted, transfer to a glass bowl.
3. Add all oils to melted butters and stir.
4. Place bowl in the refrigerator for about an hour. Once solidified, remove.

Now, gently score with a knife to make easier to mix. Add all the oils and Aloe Vera, then blend with a hand-mixer until you get the consistency you desire.

Scoop with a plastic spatula into glass jars for storage. Shelf life approx. 3 weeks.

Inspired by **Naptural85**

Clay Mask DIY

Use Glass Bowl for Mixing
[Metal bowl will weaken the power of the clay]

Cut recipe in half for shorter hair, double recipe for longer hair.

Ingredients
1 cup Rhassoul
3/4 cup Bentonite Clay
1/2 cup Kaolin Clay

1 cup Distilled Water - Room temperature
3 TBSP ACV

Oils
2 TBSP Avocado Oil
10 drops essential Lavender or Neem Oil

Apply on detangled hair (can be damp or dry)
15-30 minutes

Inspired by **Green Beauty**

For an informative explanation on the use of this clay mixture
watch this video:
https://www.youtube.com/watch?v=aP7RKfie5oQ

Cleanser DIY

African Black Soap - Single Wash Recipe

1. Purchase authentic African Black Soap made in Africa. (Check RESOURCES)
2. Cut about 1/8th of the bar (approx. 1/2 c), then cut into smaller pieces.
3. Boil/microwave 2 cups water. Let cool about 5 mins. then add cut pieces of soap.
4. Stir and let it melt - usually within 30 mins.

Once soap is liquified, add:
    10 drops Peppermint Oil
    10 drops Tea Tree Oil
    10 drops Lavender Oil
    1 tsp. Neem Oil
    1 tsp. Vitamin E
    1 tsp. Glycerin

Stir well. Let it stand for 2 hours. Then use when ready!

Inspired by **Naptural85**

Deep Conditioner DIY

1 Avocado
1 Banana - sliced in small pieces
1 TBSP. Honey
1/4 c. Aloe Vera Juice
1 tsp. Fenugreek Powder (Methi Powder)
1/4 c. Avocado Oil

Blend all ingredients into a creamy mix.
Strain in a bowl.

Apply to dry, unclean hair.
Cover with plastic cap. Leave in for 30 mins. to 1 hour.

Wash hair as usual.

DE-Tangler DIY

MIRACLE DETANGLER

Preparation ~

1-1/2 cups Water
3 TBSP. Marshmallow Root
3 TBSP. Slippery Elm
1-1/2 tsp. Grapeseed Oil
3 TBSP. Apple Cider Vinegar

Add Marshmallow Root & Slippery Elm to boiling water, let thicken for about 6-8 minutes. Take off heat. Strain in glass bowl.

Add Grapeseed Oil and ACV. Stir to mix well. Pour into squeeze bottle and apply to freshly washed hair.

Growth Masks DIY

Super-Duper Growth Mask

Mix in a glass bow.

3 TBSP Neem Oil
3 TBSP Coconut Oil
3 TBSP Amla Oil
1 TBSP Organic Honey

Put it onto your scalp and hair; massage effectively. Cover with shower cap and satin scarf. Leave in over-night.

Shampoo out the next day, continue with regular wash day routine.

From <http://hairlosscureguide.com/10-ways-you-can-use-neem-oil-for-hair-growth-to-cure-hair-loss/>

Ayurvedic Hair Mask for Conditioning

Powders

100 gm Henna
100 gm Amla
100 gm Hibiscus

Mix all powders with warm water until a paste the consistency of pancake batter.

Then add:
2 cups of moisturizing conditioner

Mix moisturizer into the batter mix until well blended.
Work in sections, smoothing the crème onto hair.
Wrap in plastic and leave on for up to 2 hours.

Rinse thoroughly with warm water, then apply leave-in conditioner. Twist or style as usual.

Growth Oil & Liquid DIY

Super-Duper Growth Oil

This oil is so potent that it is recommended to use once per week, preferably one day <u>after</u> full wash. You may modify this to suit your hair type and condition.

Preparation:

Tightly woven cheese cloth or cotton fabric cut in a single 8"x 8" square.

Fill the fabric with the following:

2 TBSP. of each of the following Ayurvedic powders
> Bhringraj
> Hibiscus
> Curry Leaves
> Amla
> Fenugreek
> Henna (optional)

Tie the powders in the fabric like a pouch. Make sure there are no holes where the powder can slip out.

In a pot, put 2 cups of water. Place pouch in the water and bring to a boil.

Boil until the water begins to turn a dark brown. When the water looks thicker in consistency, and darker brown, take away from heat and let cool. Gently press a spoon against the pouch to squeeze more of the "juice". Then remove the pouch and set pot aside.

In a cast iron Dutch-oven, over medium heat, pour 1-1/2 Cup of Sesame Oil or other high heat oil such as Grapeseed or Avocado.

While the oil is still <u>room temperature</u>, pour your powder liquid mix into the oil. Stir and mix well together. **DO NOT POUR COOL POWDER LIQUID MIX INTO HOT OIL.**

Under medium heat, bring the mixture to a boil, and allow to boil until all the "bubbles" disappear, and when you notice that the mixture is thickening and there are very few bubbles, turn off the heat. Stir and prepare to strain.

Take a glass jar, cover with cheese cloth and strain the cooled mixture into the jar. The oil can be stored for up to 90 days. Should be stored in a cool, dry, dark place until ready for use.

 Use precautions when preparing this oil. Also, perform a skin patch test to be sure you are not allergic to any of the ingredients.

Be aware that if you use Henna in this mix, your hair will over time turn reddish. If you don't want this - don't use Henna, use Cassia instead.

Fenugreek Hair Growth Oil

In a glass jar, add the following ingredients:

1 cup Coconut oil - melted
2 TBSP. Olive oil
1 TBSP. Castor Oil
2 TBSP. Henna Powder
[Use Cassia if you do not want your hair to color]
1 TBSP. Fenugreek seeds

Essential Oils:
10 drops Peppermint Oil
10 drops Rosemary Oil
10 drops Tea Tree
1/8 tsp. MSM Powder (Sulfur benefits)
1/8 tsp. Vitamin C

Stir. Allow to infuse for at least 8 hours before use and up to 4 weeks, taking what you need for use, and then discarding after 4 weeks.

Inspired by **Curly Proverbz**

Onion Massage Treatment

Preparation:
1 Yellow Onion or Red Onion finely chopped
1 Garlic cloves finely chopped
1 tsp. Cayenne Pepper

In a saucepan, add the onion and garlic cloves in 2 Cups of water.

Bring to boil. Cool.

Strain in a glass jar, and add the cayenne pepper. Stir. Store.

Best to use <u>BEFORE</u> washing your hair.

Massage gently into the scalp and around the edges, cover with plastic cap for 20-30 minutes.

Shampoo hair.

Inspired by **Green Beauty**

pH Neutralizer DIY

Helps to smooth the cuticles after washing to retain moisture.

To restore the hair's natural pH balance. This is great for HIGH porosity hair.

Apple Cider Vinegar Spritz (ACV) - pH4
    8 oz. <u>Distilled</u> Water
    1 Tsp. ACV

To learn more about the Science of ACV and pH balancing, visit **Green Beauty** on YouTube®

Protein Treatment DIY

Fermented or Boiled Rice Water

Boiled Rice Water
>1 cup of rice to 2 cups of water
>Bring to boil, strain in glass jar or spray bottle.
>
>Apply to freshly washed hair, cover with plastic cap for 20-30 minutes.
>
>Rinse out with cool water.

Fermented Rice Water (More concentrated)
>1 cup of rice to 2 cups of water in a bowl or glass jar
>Let water stand for 2 hours, drain into glass jar with lid
>
>Seal tightly and store in a dark cabinet for 2-3 days.
>
>Take the top off to reveal a "sour" smell.
>
>To stop the fermentation, refrigerate.
>
>To apply to hair, when rice water is cold, mix with room temperature water equal portions into a spray bottle. Apply to freshly washed hair. Cover with plastic cap and leave in for 20-30 minutes.
>
>Rinse out with cool water.

To understand the science of rice water on hair visit **Green Beauty** on YouTube®.

Smoothie for Hair Growth

½ Avocado
½ Banana
1 tsp. Collagen Powder (See RESOURCES)
1 tsp. of Black Seed Oil
1 tsp. of Coconut Oil
1 tsp. Flaxseeds (ground or seeds – Not oil)
Handful of Spinach, Kale, or greens of your choice
½ cup Almond Milk or your choice of liquid

Blend.

Best if you have first thing in the morning on an empty stomach.

Spritz DIY

ALOE VERA SPRITZ - Great for HIGH porosity hair.

> 8 oz. Distilled Water
> 2 TBSP. Aloe Vera Juice
> 1/4 tsp. Olive Oil
> 1/4 tsp. Leave-in Conditioner (Optional)

> Use this spritz after washing your hair to neutralize the pH and keep hair moisturized while detangling.

ROSEMARY SPRITZ - Daily Moisture

> Boil 1 pkg. of fresh rosemary sprigs in 2 cups water until sprigs turn brown or dark brown.
> Let cool. Strain into glass jar and store in refrigerator until use.
> Shelf life of approx. 14 days.

> Use this spritz twice a day to retain moisture in your hair.

HERBAL TEA SPRITZ

1/2 tsp. Lavender (crushed leaves) - Strengthens new growth hair, balances oil, relieves itching
 1/2 tsp. Sage - Adds shine and delays premature graying, stimulate growth
 1 Green Tea Bag- High in antioxidants, stimulates growth, adds shine
 1/2 tsp Bamboo Leaf Tea - High in Silica (70%), increase elasticity in the hair, reduces shedding, thickens hair strands

Boil Aloe Vera Juice, add teas, let steep 5 minutes. Cool and use massage into scalp daily.

Style Gel DIY

THE BEST DAMN FLAXSEED GEL EVER!

2 cups water in pot
Add 1/2 cup Flaxseeds
Add 1/4 cup Chia Seeds
Bring to light boil under medium heat.

Add:
1 TBSP. Slippery Elm Bark
1 TBSP. Marshmallow Root
Stir continuously. When mucus layer begins to form, remove from heat.

To keep it from thickening too much, immediately strain into a glass bowl using a metal strainer.

Let cool.

Add:
    10-15 drops of Lavender Oil
    1/4 teaspoon of Avocado Oil

Pour in glass jar, give a little shake and refrigerate until ready to use.

Will store for up to 3 weeks.

This gel is great to use for twist-outs. But is especially great for sealing in moisture after using the L.O.C. or the L.C.O. method.

Inspired by **Naptural85**

Natural RITUAL

Hair rituals are great for getting you in the habit of a routine. They are meant to be modified as needed.

The connection between my hair and the identity of who I am is so empowering.   I usually block an entire day to ensure proper care and attention to my hair. The practice has brought me to another level of inspired connection with "self" and you will find out this for yourself.

Creating your own personal hair ritual is essential for the successful hair growth and well-being of your hair. With that stated, the following ritual is one that works best **for me.**

After much trial and error, watching a gazillion videos on YouTube® and testing products on my hair over time, I created this ritual. You are free to modify and tweak this in whatever way you feel would best suit your hair needs.

Always test new products by doing a strand test or skin patch test to ensure that you do not have an allergic reaction, or can possibly cause damage to your strands.

All ingredients can be found in RESOURCES and on the website – https://hairgoalsblackbook.com

THE RITUAL

DAILY MAINTENANCE
Drink plenty of water during the day
>(Try a water app to help remind you to stay hydrated - see RESOURCES)

**Take Multi-Vitamin Supplements
**Take 1000 mg of MCM
Eat healthy, organic foods - no fried, sugar, or dairy
Spritz your hair twice a day for moisture (See RECIPES)
Sleep in a silk scarf at night or use a satin pillow case

****Do not take any supplements without first consulting your physician.**

WEEKLY
Pre-poo~
Best to do this before bedtime the day before wash day.
If you do not care to sleep mix in your hair overnight, add to your wash day routine and leave on hair at least 30 minutes.

>(3-5) 1" slices of Aloe Vera plant and 1 tbsp. Honey
>>Make sure to remove skin from Aloe Vera plant pieces. Cut into smaller pieces and put into a blender with the honey. Short pulse until all the pieces are blended thoroughly.
>>
>>Section hair and pin or twist out of the way.
>>Slather onto hair, working in each strand carefully.
>>
>>Finish with a coat of Organic Olive or Avocado Oil, or your preferred oil.
>>
>>Plastic cap, wrapped in satin scarf. Keep on overnight. Or, leave on for 30 minutes before shampoo.

Wash Day~
If pre-poo the same day as wash, rinse with warm water, then proceed.

Shampoo - African Black Soap or your favorite shampoo (See RECIPES)

Moisturizing Conditioner (No protein)

3 times a week
Fingertip massage Peppermint Oil & Water spritz
Ayurvedic Growth Oil

MONTHLY:
Refer to RECIPES and RESOURCES for products/DIYs

1st week
Clarifying Shampoo - African Black Soap
Deep Conditioner DIY
2nd week
Growth Treatment - Onion Treatment
Hot Oil Treatment - Super Duper Growth / Oil of choice
Rice Water Rinse
3rd week
Clay Mask
Protein Treatment

OTHER
Every 8 - 12 weeks
Protein Treatment using Hydrolyzed Protein - See RESOURCES

Every 4-6 months
Full Henna Treatment / Henna Mask

Natural ROUND-UP

Help Along the Way!

This natural hair journey is no joke and it takes a lot of patience, care, and knowledge. Naturals who have successfully mastered their hair game, know this to be true

The following pages introduce you to those who have been instrumental in helping me to understand my hair, communicate with it regularly, and nurture it back to its original healthy state.

You will have an opportunity to connect with these phenomenal "naturalistas" on their YouTube® channels and learn more about your own hair.

Naptural85

Green Beauty

Curly Proverbz

Power in Your Curl

22nd Century Natural Woman

NappyFu TV

Naptural85

Boho-Chic with a touch of nostalgia best describes this natural beauty.

Naptural85 (Whitney) will inspire you to take deliberate steps to nourish your hair using products from your kitchen.

Her Mango Butter Mix is off the chain! You can find a modified version in RECIPES. However, you can view her YouTube® channel for the original recipe.

If you love DIY recipes, her channel should be your first option! Her luscious locks provide evidence that going natural, in every way, is worth the effort.

Channel Handle: Naptural85
Subscribers: 877k+

FAVS
> Mango Butter Recipe (Modified version in RECIPES)

BEST ADVICE
> Keep your hair fortified with nutrients using plant-based oils and butters is important for creating "flexible" strands. It helps minimize breakage.

Green Beauty Channel

One of the most informative channels on natural hair care on YouTube®, **Green Beauty** takes learning about your natural hair to a whole other level.

When it comes to the science of how products interact with natural hair, Green Beauty demonstrates, explains, and delivers facts based on scientific proof. Never have I witnessed such in-depth explanations when it comes to the science of natural hair. This channel was instrumental in the growth, strength, and health of my hair for so many reasons. It helped me to understand how my hair type, density, and porosity would respond to the treatments being given and better tailor a ritual/regimen for me.

Every natural should tune in and watch Green Beauty -- the host and information are SUPERB!

Channel Handle: Green Beauty
Subscribers: 144k

FAVS
Real Protein Treatment (See RESOURCES)

BEST ADVICE
Stretching your hair is very important. It helps to eliminate single strand knots and aids in healthy growth.

ACV that is pH-4 is great for HIGH porosity hair because it relaxes the cuticle and aids in moisture retention.

Curly Proverbz

Adorable, beautiful, and an Ayurvedic Queen!

If you know nothing of Ayurvedic herbal treatments, you will when you check out Curly Proverbz.

Her DIY recipes use only Ayurvedic herbs, oils, and powders. She uses them in EVERYTHING! Including her own line of products, Belle Bar.

What is fascinating about **Curly Proverbz** is her natural (pun intended) magnetism. She shares a great deal of information on the use of her custom designed Ayurvedic hair care regimen as well as specifically detail any caution with its use. She helps eliminate the fear in newbies to this type of regimen.

Channel Handle: Curly Proverbz
Subscribers: 133k+

FAVS
>   Fenugreek Hair Growth Oil

BEST ADVICE
>   You don't need to do a full Henna treatment and a deep conditioner the same day. Both are strengthening, and you risk the danger of breakage and tangling. A regular conditioner after a Henna treatment will help make the hair more manageable.

Power in Your Curl

If you are not the DIY natural, and prefer to buy products because it is easier for you, **Power in Your Curl** (Kenya) is your girl!

Fresh, stylish natural beauty, are words that best describe this YouTube® Influencer.

This young lady does awesome product reviews for natural hair care products and she shares practical tips for managing your "fine" hair.

Channel Handle: Power in Your Curl
Subscribers: 43k+

FAVS
    Mielle Organics
        Babassu Oil and Mint Deep Conditioner

BEST ADVICE
    Trim hair every 3 months; best to trim yourself.

22nd Century Natural Woman

Love, love, love this Goddess!

Don't be fooled by the soft, gentle voice. This **22nd Century Natural Woman** will set you straight when it comes to natural hair care. Her regal presence commands the reverence of an African Queen. Her no nonsense regimen includes her custom developed self-named hair care line which can be found at http://www.moorket.com

Her journey is one to be admired, reaching a near length of 40" -- Beautiful locks! She really inspires naturals to set real hair goals. Simplicity, patience, and connecting to mother earth are her guiding principles. She shares great content and full processes that sometimes last up to an hour, however, well worth the watch.

Channel Handle: 22nd Century Natural Woman
Subscribers: 77k +

FAVS
> 22nd Century Natural Woman Deep Conditioner
> Hair Stew

BEST ADVICE
> Naturals with thin strands do not need to weigh the hair down with moisturizing products after a full wash.   Like heavy style creams, oils, etc. Additionally, oiling the scalp should be done sparingly or not at all after a wash day. Too much oil on the scalp will disrupt Sebum (oil) production in the scalp.

NappyFu TV

A Natural-born comedian!

NappyFu's humor is enough to watch her channel alone, but in addition she gives great advice on the care of 4C hair.

She is passionate about her 4C hair and will call-out all impersonators without hesitation.   Her specialization concerns all processes and products that enhance the health of 4C hair. She conducts intensive research and you know that she is well informed on her videos, and she wants the same for her audience.

Channel Handle: NappyFu TV
Subscribers: 150k +

FAVS
>   **All** review videos...Informative and FUNNY!

BEST ADVICE
>   You don't need a 25-step regimen to have healthy, growing hair. Stop it!

Natural
RESOURCES

Articles

Not Too Pretty - Report
A report detailing the dangers of chemicals used in the beauty industry.

https://www.ewg.org/research/not-too-pretty#.WkZ_ed-nFPZ

This report outlines the dangers of the beauty industry's most toxic chemicals and the effects it has on the body, among these are Phthalates with studies showing overwhelming evidence of reproductive damage in men and women.

10 Silicones to Avoid

https://www.naturallycurly.com/curlreading/products-ingredients/10-silicones-in-curly-hair-products-to-avoid

1. Cetearyl Methicone
2. Cetyl Dimethicone
3. Dimethicone
4. Dimethiconol
5. Stearyl Dimethicone
6. Cyclomethicone/Cyclopentasiloxane
7. Trimethylsilylamodimethicone
8. Behenoxy Dimethicone
9. Stearoxy Dimethicone
10. Amodimethicone

Names Silicones Hide Behind
https://www.naturallycurly.com/curlreading/curl-products/curlchemist-silicone-or-not-whats-in-a-name

Lipstick Alley Forums (Natural Hair Care)
https://www.lipstickalley.com/forums/natural-hair-care.546/

https://www.allure.com/gallery/13-best-hair-products-for-women-of-color

http://www.curlynikki.com/2010/09/homemade-product-recipes.html

Hair Pantry

Butters
Mango
Cocoa
Argan
Aloe Vera
Cupuacu
Tamanu
Jojoba

Clays
Rhassoul aka Ghassoul
Bentonite
Kaolin

Liquids
Apple Cider Vinegar
Glycerin
Distilled Water

Oils
Avocado Oil
Argan Oil
Coconut Oil
Sesame Oil
Neem Oil
Olive Oil
Grapeseed Oil
Black Seed Oil
Castor Oil (Hexane-free)
Jamaican Black Castor Oil (Hexane-free)
Sweet Almond Oil
Jojoba Oil
Vitamin E

Essential Oils
Peppermint
Tea Tree

Lavender
Citrus

Powders
Bhringrah
Curry Leaves
Aloe Vera
Hibiscus
Fenugreek (Methi Powder) or Seeds
Amla
Henna

Soaps
African Black Soap - Organic

Teas
Black / Green / Bamboo

Other
Honey
Fresh Rosemary
White or Brown Rice
Yellow Onions
Cayenne Pepper

Note: Powders should be stored in plastic zip-locks in the refrigerator or freezer. Additionally, any DIY products should be stored in the refrigerator for no more than 4 weeks. After 4 weeks, discard.

Recommendations

Here are some links that will connect you with natural, organic, and healthier products.

Just Natural Skincare
http://www.justnaturalskincare.com/

Green Beauty
Green Beauty offers a Hydrolyzed Wheat Protein treatment called "REAL PROTEIN TREATMENT" available in their online store at https://greenbeauty.com

CurlKit - Porosity & Density Check
http://curlkit.com/natural-hair-porosity-density/

Amazon.com
All the ingredients purchased from Amazon.com for RECIPES are found on:
https://hairgoalsblackbook.com/products

Mountain Rose Herbs
https://www.mountainroseherbs.com/ - herbs, spices, teas & DIY supplies

Felicia Leatherwood Detangling Brush
https://www.brushwiththebest.com/

GooglePlay App Store
>Water Drink Reminder

Bulk Apothecary
>https://www.bulkapothecary.com - Herbs, Oils, Whole Foods, Personal Care Products, DIY Supplies

Alodia Hair Care
>https://alodiahaircare.com/

JOURNAL & SCHEDULE

The importance of understanding your hair type will inevitably lead to your hair's condition. This can be challenging, especially since natural girls may have a diverse mix of curls on their heads.

Along with learning your curl type is the added challenge of figuring out the porosity of your hair. This indicates how much moisture your hair can handle at any given time, and what your hair does with the moisture once its attained.

Does it evaporate quickly?

Does it stay within the strands?

My hair's porosity is HIGH, but can fall in the middle sometimes, depending on the regimen/ritual performed for the week.

Without at minimum understanding of type and porosity of your hair, you can risk jeopardizing your strands. You could end up using products or doing regimens/rituals that do not favor your hair.

It is important to keep a **Hair Journal** and **Hair Schedule** (download free - see RESOURCES) to help you identify easily what is working. It will save you time and money. More importantly, it will save your hair.

The **Hair Journal** is a great place to document the products you use, DIY or store bought. It provides you with a personal feedback loop on your hair's experience with a product. Tracking your success and results can aid in better understanding what your hair likes best.

Your hair will grow best under predictable conditions. This is where the **Hair Schedule** can be handy. Plan your scheduled routines/regimens/rituals, and within 3-6 months you will notice a very visible change in your hair's behavior and health, even with minor setbacks along the way.

Your hair type may require a different approach than outlined in this book, so a little due diligence to find out what is suited for you may be required.

SCHEDULE

Download your Ritual/Regimen Tracker

http://bit.ly/hairgoalsrituals

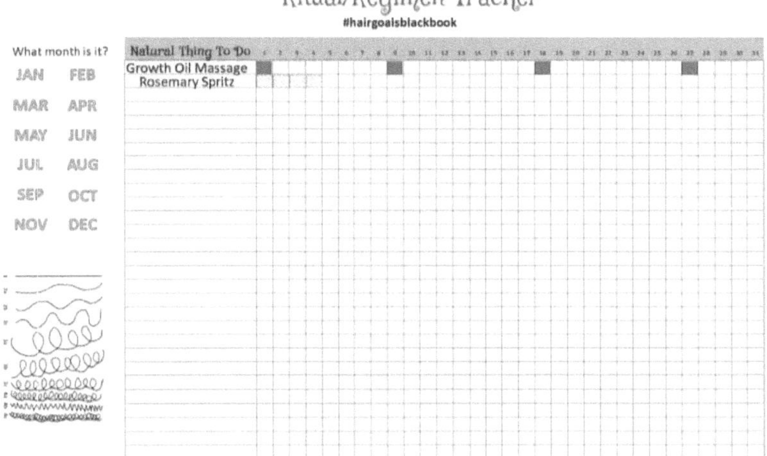

The tracker is designed to help you keep an eye on your personal hair treatment. Just circle the month, list the things or treatments you want to include in your regimen, and color or shades the dates when you will do them. There is also a handy curl pattern chart to help you determine your hair type.

JOURNAL

Your hair journey is unique, and you will have missteps, victories, and maybe even something new happen. Jot it down! You don't want to forget some of these memorable moments.

ANECDOTES

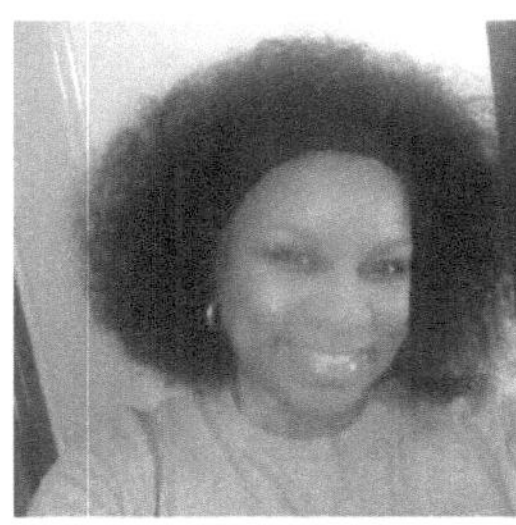

April 2013

After I cut the remaining 2" of perm from my hair, I officially started my natural journey. It was neck length, weak, and thin.

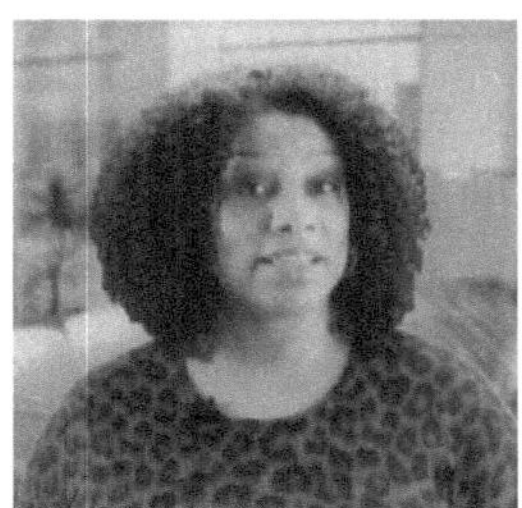

December 2016

Hair much healthier and thicker. At shoulder length with shrinkage. Curl definition much better.

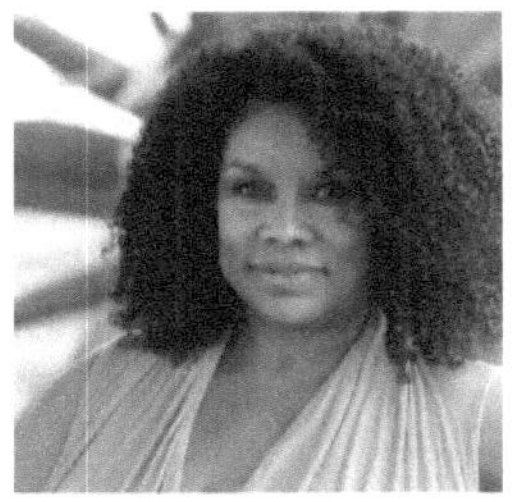

June 2017

Thicker strands due to tweaks in the regimen. Still struggling with some moisture retention issues. Ends are starting to "sit" on the shoulders.

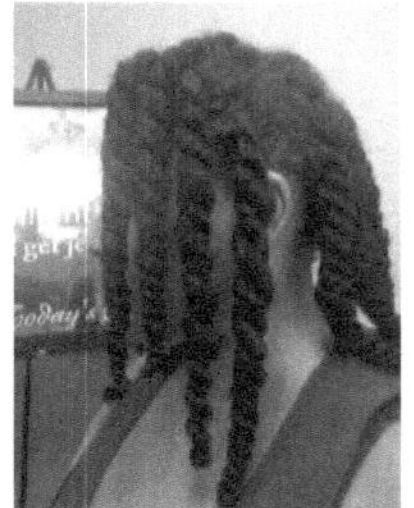

November 2017

Final tweaks in regimen in August. My hair was thicker and grew longer. This was 2 hours after a full wash routine.

As a personal note, I do not measure my hair's length like I see many do on YouTube®. For me, length is not as important as the health of my hair. If my hair is healthy, it will grow. It's that simple.

I "sweep" the ends every time I do a full wash. Sweeping is simply clipping the strands that extend longer than the rest. I do a full trim of about ¼" every six months. I don't go to salons.

Store-bought products I use are primarily curl creams.

Taliah Waajid Curly Curl Cream
Absolutely love this product. It defines the softest curls and the hold is incredible. It's a light weight cream.

Shea Moisture Curl Enhancing Smoothie
Great hold and curl definition. Not to mention, the incredible smell of this product! Delicious. It's a heavier cream.

Curls Crème Brule Whipped Curl Cream
This is a wonderful cream you can use daily for twisting or styling. Absorbs into the hair shaft. It's a lighter cream, more like a daily moisturizer cream.

TELL YOUR STORY

I would love to hear your story!

Visit the site and share your natural hair journey story or ask questions about what I talked about in this book. Let me know if this information was helpful to you, or if you have something that you discovered along the way that would help others.

hairgoalsblackbook.com

Make sure you sign up for any updates to my regimen, posted videos, or new DIY Haircare recipes.

THANK YOU FOR YOUR NATURAL BEAUTY♥

www.ingramcontent.com/pod-product-compliance
Lightning Source LLC
Chambersburg PA
CBHW031326250726
48656CB00005B/1983